CONTENTS

INTRODUCTION

Overview of the Blood Type O Diet

The Blood Type O Diet is a dietary approach that is based on the theory that individuals with blood type O should follow a specific eating plan tailored to their blood type. This diet gained popularity through the book "Eat Right for Your Type" by Dr. Peter J. D'Adamo. According to this theory, each blood type has different nutritional needs and can benefit from consuming certain foods while avoiding others.

People with blood type O are believed to have ancestral ties to hunter-gatherer populations. Therefore, the Blood Type O Diet emphasizes a high-protein, low-carbohydrate approach, reminiscent of the diet of early humans. It suggests that individuals with blood type O should consume lean proteins, fruits, vegetables, and limit or avoid grains and dairy products.

The main premise behind the Blood Type O Diet is that by following this eating plan, individuals can improve their overall health, optimize digestion, manage weight, and prevent or alleviate certain health conditions. However, it is important to note that the scientific evidence supporting this theory is limited, and more research is needed to establish its effectiveness.

Explanation of the Blood Type Theory

The Blood Type Theory, also known as the blood type

personality theory, suggests that a person's blood type is an indicator of their unique traits, characteristics, and susceptibility to certain health conditions. This theory originated in Japan with the work of Dr. Masahiko Nomi and gained further attention through Dr. Peter J. D'Adamo's book mentioned earlier.

According to this theory, each blood type (A, B, AB, and O) is associated with distinct qualities. Individuals with blood type O are often described as practical, energetic, and goal-oriented. They are believed to have a strong digestive system and thrive on high-protein diets. Blood type O individuals are thought to have evolved from ancient hunter-gatherers and are said to have a more robust immune system.

While the Blood Type Theory has gained popularity and has a significant following, it is important to note that scientific evidence supporting the specific claims made by this theory is lacking. Blood type is determined by the presence or absence of certain antigens on red blood cells, and there is currently no scientific consensus linking blood type to personality traits or specific dietary requirements.

Benefits of Following the Blood Type O Diet

Proponents of the Blood Type O Diet claim that adhering to this eating plan can provide several health benefits for individuals with blood type O. Some of the potential benefits include:

1. **Improved Digestion**: The diet emphasizes foods that are said to be well-tolerated by individuals with blood type O, such as lean meats, fruits, and vegetables. By avoiding foods that may be less compatible, it is believed that digestion can be optimized.

2. **Weight Management**: The Blood Type O Diet promotes a high-protein, low-carbohydrate approach, which may aid in weight management. Protein-rich foods are thought to enhance metabolism and promote satiety.

3. **Increased Energy**: Blood type O individuals are believed to have a naturally higher level of stomach acid, which aids in the digestion of animal proteins. By consuming a diet that aligns with their blood type, it is suggested that individuals may experience increased energy levels.

4. **Reduced Inflammation**: The diet recommends avoiding certain foods, such as grains and dairy products, which are thought to cause inflammation in individuals with blood type O. By following the prescribed diet, proponents claim that inflammation can be reduced.

5. **Disease Prevention**: Advocates of the Blood Type O Diet argue that adhering to this eating plan can lower the risk of certain health conditions, including cardiovascular disease and certain types of cancer. However, it is essential to note that more scientific research is needed to substantiate these claims.

Purpose and Goals of the Ebook

The purpose of the Ebook is to provide comprehensive information and guidance on the Blood Type O Diet. It aims to educate readers about the theory behind the diet, the recommended foods, and the potential benefits associated with following this eating plan.

The goals of the Ebook include:

1. **Informing Readers**: The Ebook intends to provide a clear and concise overview of the Blood Type O Diet, explaining the theory, its origins, and how it relates to blood type O individuals.

2. **Exploring the Science**: While the scientific evidence supporting the Blood Type Theory is limited, the Ebook can present the existing research and offer an objective perspective on the topic.

3. **Providing Practical Guidance**: The Ebook will offer practical advice on how to implement the Blood Type O Diet, including meal planning, recipe suggestions, and tips for dining out.

4. **Addressing Potential Concerns**: The Ebook will address common concerns or criticisms regarding the Blood Type O Diet, providing a balanced view of the topic and allowing readers to make informed decisions.

5. **Empowering Readers**: Ultimately, the Ebook aims to empower readers to make dietary choices that align with their individual needs and preferences. It will encourage critical thinking and highlight the importance of personalized nutrition.

In conclusion, the Blood Type O Diet is a dietary approach that suggests individuals with blood type O should follow a specific eating plan tailored to their blood type. While it has gained popularity, the scientific evidence supporting this theory is limited. The Ebook aims to provide a comprehensive guide to the Blood Type O Diet, offering information, practical advice, and addressing potential concerns to empower readers in making informed decisions about their dietary choices.

UNDERSTANDING BLOOD TYPE O

Description of Blood Type O

Blood type O is one of the four main blood types, along with A, B, and AB. It is the most common blood type globally, with approximately 45% of the world's population belonging to this group. Blood type is determined by the presence or absence of specific antigens on the surface of red blood cells.

Individuals with blood type O have red blood cells that do not have A or B antigens. However, they do have both A and B antibodies in their plasma. This means that if a person with blood type O receives a blood transfusion from someone with types A, B, or AB, their immune system may recognize the transfused blood as foreign and mount an immune response.

In terms of blood type compatibility for donations, people with blood type O are considered universal donors, as their blood can be given to individuals with any blood type. However, individuals with blood type O can only receive blood from other type O individuals.

Characteristics and Traits of People with Blood Type O

According to the Blood Type Theory, individuals with

blood type O are associated with specific characteristics and traits. It is important to note that while these associations exist in the theory, scientific evidence supporting them is currently limited and inconclusive. Nevertheless, here are some common characteristics often attributed to people with blood type O:

1. **Energetic and Active**: Blood type O individuals are often described as energetic, lively, and active. They are believed to have a natural inclination towards physical activities and exercise.

2. **Goal-Oriented**: Individuals with blood type O are said to be goal-oriented and focused. They are often determined and strive to achieve their objectives.

3. **Strong-willed**: People with blood type O are believed to be strong-willed and assertive. They tend to be decisive and assert their opinions.

4. **Practical and Realistic**: Blood type O individuals are often considered practical and down-to-earth. They tend to have a realistic perspective and approach to life.

5. **Optimistic**: Individuals with blood type O are said to have an optimistic outlook. They are often described as positive thinkers and have a resilient nature.

6. **Strong Digestive System**: Blood type O individuals are believed to have a robust digestive system. They are thought to metabolize animal proteins efficiently.

Again, it is crucial to emphasize that the associations between blood type and personality traits are based on the

Blood Type Theory and lack substantial scientific evidence.

Health Considerations for Blood Type O Individuals

While the Blood Type O Diet suggests specific dietary recommendations for blood type O individuals, it is important to remember that individual variations and overall health status should also be taken into account. Here are some general health considerations for individuals with blood type O:

1. **Dietary Recommendations**: The Blood Type O Diet emphasizes a high-protein, low-carbohydrate approach. It suggests consuming lean meats, fish, fruits, and vegetables, while limiting or avoiding grains and dairy products. However, it is essential to consult with a healthcare professional or registered dietitian before making significant dietary changes.

2. **Exercise Routine**: Blood type O individuals are often encouraged to engage in regular physical activity and exercise. Activities such as cardio exercises, strength training, and high-intensity workouts are typically recommended.

3. **Stress Management**: People with blood type O are believed to have a higher level of cortisol, a stress hormone. It is important for blood type O individuals to manage stress effectively through relaxation techniques, mindfulness practices, or engaging in hobbies and activities that help reduce stress levels.

4. **Health Conditions**: While blood type does not determine a person's susceptibility to specific health conditions, some studies have suggested

that blood type O individuals may have a slightly lower risk of developing certain diseases such as pancreatic cancer and certain cardiovascular conditions. However, more research is needed to confirm these findings.

5. **Individualized Approach**: It is crucial for blood type O individuals, like anyone else, to adopt an individualized approach to their health. Factors such as age, gender, genetics, lifestyle, and overall health should be considered when making decisions about diet, exercise, and healthcare.

It is important to approach the associations between blood type and health or personality traits with caution. While the Blood Type Theory suggests certain connections, scientific evidence supporting these claims is currently limited. Individual variations and overall health should be the primary factors considered when making lifestyle and healthcare decisions. Consulting with a healthcare professional or registered dietitian can provide personalized guidance and support.

THE SCIENCE BEHIND THE BLOOD TYPE O DIET

Explanation of the Blood Type Theory

The Blood Type Theory suggests that an individual's blood type can influence various aspects of their health, including digestion, metabolism, and susceptibility to certain diseases. This theory was popularized by Dr. Peter J. D'Adamo in his book "Eat Right for Your Type."

According to the Blood Type Theory, different blood types (A, B, AB, and O) evolved at different points in human history and are associated with different dietary needs. The theory suggests that each blood type has specific antigens that interact with different foods, affecting digestion and overall health.

The Blood Type Theory proposes that blood type O individuals, who are believed to have ancestral ties to hunter-gatherer populations, should follow a high-protein, low-carbohydrate diet. It suggests that this type of diet aligns with the genetic makeup of blood type O individuals and optimizes their health.

While the Blood Type Theory has gained popularity, it is important to note that scientific evidence supporting the specific claims made by this theory is limited. The associations between blood type and dietary recommendations require further research and validation.

How Blood Type O Affects Digestion and Metabolism

According to the Blood Type Theory, blood type O individuals have a unique digestive system and metabolism. They are believed to have a higher level of stomach acid and enzyme production, which aids in the efficient digestion of animal proteins.

Blood type O individuals are thought to thrive on a diet rich in lean meats, fish, and poultry. These protein sources are believed to be more easily digested and utilized by their bodies. Additionally, the theory suggests that blood type O individuals have a more efficient metabolism for breaking down and using fats.

The recommended high-protein, low-carbohydrate diet for blood type O is said to support their natural metabolic tendencies and promote weight management. However, it is important to note that individual variations in metabolism exist, and not all blood type O individuals will have identical responses to the same dietary approach.

Impact of Blood Type O on Nutrient Absorption

The Blood Type Theory suggests that blood type O individuals may have specific nutrient absorption characteristics influenced by their blood type. For example, it is believed that blood type O individuals have a more efficient ability to absorb and utilize iron from animal sources.

Additionally, the theory suggests that blood type O individuals may have a reduced ability to digest and absorb certain carbohydrates found in grains and legumes. This is said to be due to the lower levels of specific enzymes related to carbohydrate metabolism.

However, it is important to note that the impact of blood type on nutrient absorption is still an area of ongoing research. The individual variations in gut microbiota, genetic factors, and overall health can also influence nutrient absorption and utilization.

Research and Studies Supporting the Blood Type O Diet

The scientific research supporting the Blood Type O Diet is limited and has produced mixed results. While some studies have suggested potential health benefits associated with following a diet aligned with blood type O, other studies have not found significant correlations.

For example, a small study published in the journal "The American Journal of Clinical Nutrition" found that blood type O individuals may have a lower risk of developing heart disease compared to individuals with other blood types. However, more extensive and well-controlled studies are needed to confirm these findings.

Another study published in the "Journal of Human Nutrition and Dietetics" examined the effects of the Blood Type Diet on various health markers. The study found that adherence to the Blood Type O Diet was associated with improvements in certain cardiovascular risk factors, such as blood pressure and cholesterol levels. However, this study had limitations, including a small sample size and self-reported dietary data.

It is important to approach the research supporting the Blood Type O Diet with caution and critically evaluate the methodology and findings of each study. More high-quality, large-scale studies are needed to establish the effectiveness and validity of this dietary approach.

In conclusion, the Blood Type Theory suggests that blood type O individuals have specific dietary needs and metabolic characteristics. The theory proposes a high-protein, low-carbohydrate diet for blood type O individuals. However, the scientific evidence supporting the Blood Type O Diet is limited and inconclusive. Individual variations, overall health, and personal preferences should be taken into account when making dietary choices. Consulting with a healthcare professional or registered dietitian can provide personalized guidance and support.

FOOD RECOMMENDATIONS FOR BLOOD TYPE O

General Guidelines for Blood Type O Individuals

For individuals with blood type O, the Blood Type O Diet suggests the following general guidelines to support overall health and well-being:

1. **Focus on Whole Foods**: Emphasize whole, unprocessed foods in your diet. Opt for fresh fruits, vegetables, lean meats, and fish.

2. **Stay Hydrated**: Drink an adequate amount of water throughout the day to maintain hydration.

3. **Regular Physical Activity**: Engage in regular physical activity and exercise to support overall health and maintain a healthy weight.

4. **Manage Stress**: Implement stress management techniques such as meditation, yoga, or deep breathing exercises to reduce stress levels.

5. **Get Sufficient Sleep**: Aim for a consistent sleep

schedule and prioritize getting enough sleep to support optimal health.

6. **Consult a Healthcare Professional**: It is recommended to consult with a healthcare professional or registered dietitian before making significant changes to your diet or lifestyle.

Foods to Emphasize in the Blood Type O Diet

The Blood Type O Diet suggests that individuals with blood type O should focus on the following types of foods:

1. High-Protein Sources

Blood type O individuals are encouraged to include ample amounts of lean meats and poultry in their diet. Good protein sources for blood type O include:

- Lean beef
- Lamb
- Venison
- Turkey
- Chicken

It is advisable to choose lean cuts of meat and remove visible fat before cooking. Grilling, baking, or broiling meats is preferred over frying.

2. Fruits and Vegetables

Blood type O individuals are advised to consume a variety of fruits and vegetables, focusing on antioxidant-rich options. Some recommended choices include:

- Kale
- Spinach
- Broccoli

- Onions
- Berries (blueberries, strawberries, etc.)
- Cherries
- Plums
- Prunes

These fruits and vegetables provide essential vitamins, minerals, and antioxidants that can support overall health.

3. Healthy Fats and Oils

In the Blood Type O Diet, healthy fats and oils are considered beneficial. Some examples include:

- Olive oil
- Flaxseed oil
- Avocado
- Walnuts
- Almonds
- Hazelnuts

These sources of healthy fats can provide essential fatty acids and contribute to a balanced diet.

Foods to Avoid or Limit in the Blood Type O Diet

The Blood Type O Diet suggests that individuals with blood type O should avoid or limit certain types of foods that may not be compatible with their blood type. These include:

1. Grains and Gluten

Grains, especially those containing gluten, are often recommended to be avoided or limited in the Blood Type O Diet. Some examples include:

- Wheat

- Barley
- Rye
- Bulgur
- Corn

These grains are believed to be less compatible with the digestive system of blood type O individuals.

2. Dairy Products

Dairy products are generally advised to be limited in the Blood Type O Diet. This includes:

- Milk
- Cheese
- Yogurt
- Butter

Blood type O individuals are encouraged to explore alternative options such as nut-based milk or dairy-free alternatives.

3. Legumes and Beans

Legumes and beans are typically restricted in the Blood Type O Diet. Examples include:

- Kidney beans
- Navy beans
- Lentils
- Chickpeas

These foods are believed to have lectins that may be less compatible with blood type O individuals.

It is important to remember that individual variations

exist, and not all blood type O individuals may have the same reactions to specific foods. Consulting with a healthcare professional or registered dietitian is advisable to personalize dietary recommendations and ensure nutritional adequacy.

MEAL PLANNING FOR BLOOD TYPE O INDIVIDUALS

Sample Meal Plan for a Typical Day

Here is a sample meal plan for a typical day following the Blood Type O Diet:

Breakfast:

- Scrambled eggs with vegetables (such as spinach, bell peppers, and onions)
- A side of fresh fruit (such as berries or a grapefruit)

Mid-Morning Snack:

- Handful of almonds or walnuts

Lunch:

- Grilled chicken breast or turkey breast
- A mixed salad with leafy greens, tomatoes, cucumbers, and olive oil dressing
- Steamed broccoli or asparagus on the side

Afternoon Snack:

- Sliced apple with almond butter

Dinner:

- Grilled salmon or lean beef steak
- Steamed kale or spinach
- Quinoa or brown rice (optional)

Evening Snack:

- Carrot sticks with hummus

Recipe Ideas and Suggestions for Blood Type O

Here are some recipe ideas and suggestions to incorporate into the Blood Type O Diet:

1. Grilled Lemon Herb Chicken: Marinate chicken breasts in a mixture of lemon juice, olive oil, garlic, and herbs. Grill until cooked through and serve with a side of steamed vegetables.

2. Baked Salmon with Roasted Vegetables: Season salmon fillets with herbs, lemon zest, and olive oil. Bake in the oven and serve with roasted Brussels sprouts, bell peppers, and onions.

3. Stir-Fried Beef with Vegetables: Sauté lean beef strips with garlic, ginger, and soy sauce. Add a variety of stir-fry vegetables like broccoli, bell peppers, and mushrooms. Serve over a bed of cauliflower rice.

4. Quinoa Salad with Avocado and Chicken: Combine cooked quinoa with diced avocado, cherry tomatoes, grilled chicken, and a squeeze of lemon juice. Toss with olive oil and fresh herbs for a nutritious and filling salad.

5. Turkey Lettuce Wraps: Sauté ground turkey with onions, garlic, and your choice of vegetables. Serve the mixture in lettuce cups for a light and satisfying meal.

Tips for Dining Out and Social Situations

Navigating dining out and social situations while following the Blood Type O Diet can be manageable with these tips:

1. **Research Restaurants**: Look up the menu and options beforehand to find restaurants that offer suitable choices for your dietary needs.

2. **Customize Your Order**: Don't hesitate to request modifications to your meal. Ask for lean meats, steamed or grilled vegetables, and salad options without dressings or with olive oil-based dressings.

3. **Communicate with Waitstaff**: Inform your server about any dietary restrictions or preferences. They may be able to provide recommendations or accommodate your needs.

4. **Choose Wisely**: Opt for protein-rich dishes such as grilled chicken, fish, or lean beef, paired with vegetables. Avoid fried and breaded options.

5. **Be Mindful of Sauces and Dressings**: Request dressings and sauces on the side to control the amount you consume. Avoid creamy or high-sugar options and opt for simple vinaigrettes or olive oil.

6. **Focus on Company**: Remember that social situations are about more than just food. Enjoy the company of friends and loved ones, and don't let dietary restrictions overshadow the experience.

Remember, the Blood Type O Diet is a personal choice, and individual variations may exist. It is important to listen to your body, make informed choices, and consult with a healthcare professional or registered dietitian for personalized guidance.

LIFESTYLE RECOMMENDATIONS FOR BLOOD TYPE O

Exercise and Physical Activity for Blood Type O

Regular exercise and physical activity play a crucial role in maintaining good health for individuals with blood type O. This blood type is believed to have evolved from ancient hunter-gatherers who were physically active and relied heavily on high-intensity activities. Engaging in suitable exercises can help blood type O individuals optimize their overall well-being and manage weight effectively. Here are some exercise and physical activity recommendations specifically tailored for individuals with blood type O:

1. **Cardiovascular Exercises**: Blood type O individuals tend to have higher levels of adrenaline and a more robust cardiovascular system. Therefore, activities that elevate the heart rate and improve cardiovascular health are beneficial. These can include brisk walking, jogging, cycling, swimming, and high-intensity interval training (HIIT).

2. **Strength Training**: Incorporating strength training exercises into the workout routine can be highly advantageous for blood type O individuals. It helps in building and maintaining lean muscle mass, which boosts metabolism and contributes to weight management. Resistance training using free weights, machines, or bodyweight exercises like push-ups, squats, and lunges are recommended.

3. **Functional Exercises**: Blood type O individuals often thrive in activities that mimic their ancestors' hunter-gatherer lifestyle. Functional exercises such as kettlebell swings, burpees, battle ropes, and agility drills can improve strength, endurance, and overall functional fitness.

4. **Mind-Body Exercises**: Stress management is particularly important for blood type O individuals, and mind-body exercises can be highly beneficial in achieving this. Practices like yoga, tai chi, and Pilates not only enhance flexibility and balance but also promote relaxation, mindfulness, and emotional well-being.

5. **Outdoor Activities**: Spending time in nature can have a profound impact on the physical and mental health of blood type O individuals. Outdoor activities like hiking, trail running, rock climbing, and team sports can provide both exercise and the therapeutic benefits of being in a natural environment.

Remember to consult with a healthcare professional or certified fitness trainer before starting any new exercise regimen, especially if you have any underlying medical conditions. Tailor your workouts to your fitness level, gradually increasing intensity and duration over time. Listen to your body and modify exercises as needed to prevent injury and ensure a safe and enjoyable fitness journey.

Stress Management Techniques

Stress is an inevitable part of life, but effective stress management techniques can help individuals with blood type O maintain a healthy balance and reduce the negative impact of stress on their well-being. Here are some strategies that can assist blood type O individuals in managing stress effectively:

1. **Physical Activity**: Engaging in regular physical activity is not only beneficial for physical health but also serves as a powerful stress management tool. Exercise releases endorphins, the body's natural mood boosters, and reduces the production of stress hormones. Find activities that you enjoy and incorporate them into your daily routine.

2. **Mindfulness and Meditation**: Practicing mindfulness and meditation techniques can significantly reduce stress levels. Deep breathing exercises, progressive muscle relaxation, and guided imagery are effective tools for calming the mind and promoting relaxation. Dedicate a few minutes each day to these practices to experience their benefits.

3. **Time Management**: Blood type O individuals often have a strong sense of responsibility and can become overwhelmed by taking on too

much. Learning effective time management skills, setting priorities, and delegating tasks can help alleviate stress and create a better work-life balance.

4. **Social Support**: Cultivating strong social connections and seeking support from friends and family can provide a valuable outlet for stress. Sharing concerns, seeking advice, or simply spending quality time with loved ones can help individuals with blood type O feel supported and better equipped to deal with stress.

5. **Healthy Lifestyle Habits**: Adopting a healthy lifestyle is crucial for managing stress. Ensure you are getting adequate sleep, maintaining a balanced diet, and avoiding excessive caffeine and alcohol intake. These lifestyle factors can significantly impact your stress levels and overall well-being.

6. **Hobbies and Relaxation Techniques**: Engaging in hobbies and activities that bring joy and relaxation can help counteract the effects of stress. Whether it's reading, listening to music, painting, gardening, or any other activity that brings you peace and happiness, make time for these pursuits regularly.

Remember that everyone's response to stress is unique, so it's essential to explore and identify what techniques work best for you. Experiment with different strategies and observe their effects on your stress levels. If chronic stress persists or becomes unmanageable, consider seeking professional help from a therapist or counselor.

Sleep and Rest Guidelines for Blood Type O Individuals

Adequate sleep and rest are crucial for overall health and well-being, especially for individuals with blood type O. Quality sleep supports optimal physical and mental functioning, helps regulate hormone levels, and promotes a strong immune system. Here are some sleep and rest guidelines specifically tailored for blood type O individuals:

1. **Establish a Consistent Sleep Schedule**: Aim to go to bed and wake up at the same time each day, even on weekends. This helps regulate the body's internal clock and promotes better sleep quality. Create a relaxing bedtime routine to signal your body that it's time to wind down.

2. **Create a Sleep-Friendly Environment**: Make your bedroom a sanctuary for sleep. Ensure the room is dark, quiet, and at a comfortable temperature. Remove electronic devices or use blue light filters to minimize exposure to stimulating screens before bedtime. Invest in a supportive mattress and pillow that suit your preferences.

3. **Manage Stress Before Bed**: Blood type O individuals can be prone to overthinking and excessive mental stimulation, which can interfere with sleep. Practice stress management techniques, such as deep breathing exercises or journaling, to calm the mind before bedtime. Consider creating a to-do list for the next day to alleviate worries about forgetting important tasks.

4. **Limit Stimulants and Heavy Meals**: Avoid

consuming stimulants like caffeine and nicotine in the evening, as they can disrupt sleep patterns. Additionally, consuming heavy meals close to bedtime can cause discomfort and indigestion, making it harder to fall asleep. Opt for light, easily digestible snacks if needed.

5. **Create a Sleep-Conducive Routine**: Engage in relaxing activities before bed to prepare your mind and body for sleep. This can include reading a book, taking a warm bath, practicing gentle stretching or yoga, or listening to calming music. Avoid stimulating activities or bright lights that can interfere with the natural sleep-wake cycle.

6. **Limit Napping**: While a short power nap can be rejuvenating, excessive daytime napping can disrupt nighttime sleep. If you feel the need to nap, keep it brief (around 20-30 minutes) and avoid napping too close to your bedtime.

Prioritize sleep and make it a non-negotiable part of your daily routine. If you consistently struggle with sleep issues or suspect you may have a sleep disorder, consult with a healthcare professional for further evaluation and guidance.

Supplement Suggestions for Blood Type O

Supplements can complement a balanced diet and provide additional support to individuals with blood type O. Although obtaining nutrients from whole foods should be the primary focus, certain supplements may be beneficial for blood type O individuals. Here are some supplement suggestions to consider:

1. **Digestive Enzymes**: Blood type O individuals

often have lower levels of stomach acid and reduced ability to digest certain foods. Digestive enzyme supplements, particularly those containing protease, can support the breakdown and absorption of proteins, promoting better digestion and nutrient utilization.

2. **Probiotics**: A healthy gut is essential for overall well-being. Probiotic supplements can help maintain a balanced gut microbiome and support digestive health. Look for a high-quality probiotic formula with strains specifically beneficial for blood type O individuals.

3. **Vitamin D**: Blood type O individuals tend to have lower vitamin D levels, especially if they live in regions with limited sunlight exposure. Consider taking a vitamin D supplement to support bone health, immune function, and overall vitality. Consult with a healthcare professional to determine the appropriate dosage.

4. **Essential Fatty Acids**: Omega-3 fatty acids, such as those found in fish oil supplements, provide numerous health benefits, including reducing inflammation and supporting heart health. Blood type O individuals may benefit from incorporating omega-3 supplements into their diet, particularly if they don't consume fatty fish regularly.

5. **Herbal Supplements**: Certain herbal supplements can support specific health needs of blood type O individuals. For example, green tea extract may aid in weight management and provide antioxidant benefits, while turmeric supplements

can help reduce inflammation. Always consult with a healthcare professional before starting any herbal supplements.

Remember, supplements should not replace a balanced diet but rather complement it. It's crucial to consult with a healthcare professional or registered dietitian before starting any new supplements to ensure they are appropriate for your individual needs and do not interfere with any existing medications or conditions.

In conclusion, incorporating regular exercise, managing stress effectively, prioritizing sleep, and considering appropriate supplements can significantly contribute to the overall well-being of individuals with blood type O. By adopting these recommendations and making them a part of a holistic lifestyle, blood type O individuals can optimize their health and lead vibrant, energetic lives.

RECIPES FOR BLOOD TYPE O

Grilled Chicken Breast with Steamed Broccoli and Quinoa

Description: This flavorful and nutritious meal features tender grilled chicken breast accompanied by steamed broccoli and quinoa. It's a perfect combination of lean protein, fiber-rich vegetables, and a hearty grain.

Ingredients:

- 4 boneless, skinless chicken breasts
- 2 cups broccoli florets
- 1 cup quinoa
- 2 tablespoons olive oil
- Salt and pepper to taste
- Optional: lemon wedges for serving

Instructions:

1. Preheat the grill to medium-high heat.

2. Season the chicken breasts with salt and pepper on both sides.

3. Grill the chicken for about 6-8 minutes per side or until cooked through and no longer pink in the center. Set aside to rest.

4. In the meantime, prepare the quinoa according to the package instructions.

5. Steam the broccoli until tender yet crisp, about 5 minutes.

6. Heat olive oil in a pan over medium heat and sauté the steamed broccoli for 2-3 minutes.

7. Divide the cooked quinoa onto plates, top with grilled chicken breasts, and serve with sautéed broccoli on the side.

8. Optional: Squeeze fresh lemon juice over the chicken for added zest.

Nutritional Information:

- Calories: 350
- Protein: 40g
- Carbohydrates: 30g
- Fat: 10g
- Fiber: 5g

Stir-Fried Beef with Bell Peppers and Brown Rice

Description: This savory stir-fry combines tender beef, vibrant bell peppers, and wholesome brown rice. It's a quick and delicious meal packed with flavors and essential nutrients.

Ingredients:

- 1 pound beef sirloin, thinly sliced
- 2 bell peppers (assorted colors), thinly sliced
- 1 cup cooked brown rice

- 3 tablespoons soy sauce

- 2 tablespoons sesame oil

- 2 cloves garlic, minced

- 1 teaspoon ginger, grated

- Salt and pepper to taste

- Optional: sliced green onions for garnish

Instructions:

1. Heat sesame oil in a large skillet or wok over medium-high heat.

2. Add minced garlic and grated ginger, and sauté for 1 minute until fragrant.

3. Add the beef slices and stir-fry for 2-3 minutes until browned.

4. Add the sliced bell peppers and continue to stir-fry for an additional 2 minutes until the peppers are tender-crisp.

5. Pour in the soy sauce and season with salt and pepper to taste. Stir well to coat the ingredients evenly.

6. Reduce the heat to low and simmer for another 2 minutes.

7. Serve the stir-fried beef and bell peppers over a bed of cooked brown rice.

8. Optional: Garnish with sliced green onions for added freshness.

Nutritional Information:

- Calories: 400

- Protein: 25g

- Carbohydrates: 35g

- Fat: 18g

- Fiber: 6g

Baked Salmon with Roasted Asparagus and Sweet Potato

Description: This wholesome meal features succulent baked salmon alongside roasted asparagus and sweet potato. It's a delightful combination of flavors that provides a nourishing boost of omega-3 fatty acids, vitamins, and minerals.

Ingredients:

- 4 salmon fillets

- 1 bunch asparagus, trimmed

- 2 medium sweet potatoes, peeled and cubed

- 2 tablespoons olive oil

- 1 teaspoon garlic powder

- 1 teaspoon dried dill

- Salt and pepper to taste

- Optional: lemon wedges for serving

Instructions:

1. Preheat the oven to 400°F (200°C) and line a baking sheet with parchment paper.

2. Place the salmon fillets, asparagus spears, and cubed sweet potatoes on the prepared baking sheet.

3. Drizzle olive oil over the ingredients and sprinkle

with garlic powder, dried dill, salt, and pepper.

4. Toss everything together to coat evenly with the seasonings and oil.

5. Bake in the preheated oven for 12-15 minutes, or until the salmon is cooked through and flakes easily with a fork.

6. Remove from the oven and let it rest for a few minutes.

7. Serve the baked salmon with roasted asparagus and sweet potato.

8. Optional: Squeeze fresh lemon juice over the salmon for a burst of citrus flavor.

Nutritional Information:

- Calories: 450
- Protein: 30g
- Carbohydrates: 30g
- Fat: 22g
- Fiber: 6g

Turkey Chili with Mixed Vegetables

Description: This hearty turkey chili is loaded with a variety of mixed vegetables, creating a nutritious and comforting meal. Packed with protein and fiber, it's a satisfying dish that will warm you up from the inside out.

Ingredients:

- 1 pound ground turkey
- 1 onion, diced
- 2 cloves garlic, minced

- 1 bell pepper, diced
- 1 zucchini, diced
- 1 cup corn kernels
- 1 can (15 ounces) kidney beans, rinsed and drained
- 1 can (15 ounces) diced tomatoes
- 2 tablespoons tomato paste
- 2 teaspoons chili powder
- 1 teaspoon cumin
- Salt and pepper to taste
- Optional toppings: shredded cheese, chopped cilantro, sour cream

Instructions:

1. In a large pot or Dutch oven, heat some oil over medium heat.
2. Add the diced onion and minced garlic, and sauté until fragrant and translucent.
3. Add the ground turkey and cook until browned, breaking it up with a spoon.
4. Add the diced bell pepper, zucchini, corn kernels, kidney beans, diced tomatoes, tomato paste, chili powder, cumin, salt, and pepper. Stir well to combine.
5. Bring the chili to a simmer, then reduce the heat to low. Cover and let it cook for about 30 minutes, stirring occasionally.
6. Taste and adjust the seasonings if needed.

7. Serve the turkey chili hot, garnished with shredded cheese, chopped cilantro, and a dollop of sour cream, if desired.

Nutritional Information:

- Calories: 350
- Protein: 25g
- Carbohydrates: 30g
- Fat: 12g
- Fiber: 8g

Shrimp and Vegetable Stir-Fry with Cauliflower Rice

Description: This light and flavorful shrimp stir-fry is paired with colorful vegetables and cauliflower rice for a low-carb, gluten-free option. It's a quick and healthy meal that's bursting with fresh flavors.

Ingredients:

- 1 pound shrimp, peeled and deveined
- 2 tablespoons soy sauce
- 1 tablespoon sesame oil
- 1 tablespoon minced ginger
- 2 cloves garlic, minced
- 1 bell pepper, thinly sliced
- 1 cup snap peas
- 1 carrot, julienned
- 1 head cauliflower, riced
- 2 green onions, sliced

- Salt and pepper to taste

- Optional: sesame seeds for garnish

Instructions:

1. In a small bowl, combine soy sauce, sesame oil, minced ginger, and minced garlic. Set aside.

2. Heat a large skillet or wok over medium-high heat.

3. Add the shrimp and stir-fry for 2-3 minutes until pink and cooked through. Remove from the skillet and set aside.

4. In the same skillet, add the sliced bell pepper, snap peas, and julienned carrot. Stir-fry for 3-4 minutes until the vegetables are crisp-tender.

5. Push the vegetables to one side of the skillet and add the cauliflower rice to the other side. Cook for 2-3 minutes, stirring occasionally, until the cauliflower is tender.

6. Return the shrimp to the skillet and pour the sauce over the ingredients. Stir well to coat everything evenly. Cook for an additional 1-2 minutes to heat through.

7. Season with salt and pepper to taste.

8. Serve the shrimp and vegetable stir-fry with cauliflower rice, garnished with sliced green onions and sesame seeds.

Nutritional Information:

- Calories: 250

- Protein: 25g

- Carbohydrates: 15g

- Fat: 10g

- Fiber: 5g

Grilled Lean Steak with Sautéed Spinach and Roasted Butternut Squash

Description: Indulge in a satisfying meal with this grilled lean steak accompanied by sautéed spinach and roasted butternut squash. It's a protein-packed dish complemented by nutritious greens and sweet roasted squash.

Ingredients:

- 2 lean steak cuts (such as sirloin or flank steak)

- 4 cups fresh spinach leaves

- 1 small butternut squash, peeled, seeded, and cubed

- 2 tablespoons olive oil

- 2 cloves garlic, minced

- Salt and pepper to taste

- Optional: balsamic glaze for drizzling

Instructions:

1. Preheat the grill to medium-high heat.

2. Rub the steaks with olive oil and season with salt and pepper.

3. Grill the steaks for 4-6 minutes per side, or until desired doneness. Remove from the grill and let them rest for a few minutes before slicing.

4. Meanwhile, preheat the oven to 400°F (200°C).

5. In a large bowl, toss the cubed butternut squash

with olive oil, minced garlic, salt, and pepper.

6. Spread the squash in a single layer on a baking sheet and roast for 20-25 minutes until tender and lightly browned.

7. In a separate pan, heat some olive oil over medium heat. Add the spinach leaves and sauté for 2-3 minutes until wilted.

8. Slice the grilled steak and serve it alongside sautéed spinach and roasted butternut squash.

9. Optional: Drizzle with balsamic glaze for added flavor.

Nutritional Information:

- Calories: 400
- Protein: 35g
- Carbohydrates: 20g
- Fat: 18g
- Fiber: 5g

Tuna Salad with Mixed Greens and Avocado

Description: This refreshing tuna salad combines tender mixed greens, protein-rich tuna, and creamy avocado. It's a light and satisfying dish that's perfect for a quick and healthy meal.

Ingredients:

- 2 cans (5 ounces each) tuna, drained
- 4 cups mixed greens
- 1 avocado, diced
- 1/2 cucumber, sliced

- 1/4 red onion, thinly sliced
- 1/4 cup cherry tomatoes, halved
- 2 tablespoons lemon juice
- 2 tablespoons olive oil
- Salt and pepper to taste

Instructions:

1. In a large bowl, combine the drained tuna, mixed greens, diced avocado, cucumber slices, red onion slices, and cherry tomato halves.

2. In a small bowl, whisk together the lemon juice, olive oil, salt, and pepper to make the dressing.

3. Drizzle the dressing over the tuna salad and toss gently to coat all the ingredients.

4. Serve the tuna salad chilled and enjoy!

Nutritional Information:

- Calories: 300
- Protein: 25g
- Carbohydrates: 10g
- Fat: 18g
- Fiber: 6g

Chicken Fajita Bowl with Lettuce, Tomatoes, and Guacamole

Description: This flavorful chicken fajita bowl is packed with seasoned chicken, crisp lettuce, juicy tomatoes, and creamy guacamole. It's a satisfying and healthy option for a delicious Tex-Mex-inspired meal.

Ingredients:

- 2 chicken breasts, sliced
- 1 bell pepper, sliced
- 1 onion, sliced
- 2 tablespoons fajita seasoning
- 4 cups lettuce, shredded
- 1 cup cherry tomatoes, halved
- 1 avocado, diced
- Juice of 1 lime
- Salt and pepper to taste

Instructions:

1. Heat some oil in a skillet over medium heat. Add the sliced chicken and cook until browned and cooked through.

2. Remove the chicken from the skillet and set it aside.

3. In the same skillet, add the sliced bell pepper and onion. Cook until they are tender and slightly charred.

4. Return the cooked chicken to the skillet and sprinkle fajita seasoning over the ingredients. Stir well to coat everything evenly.

5. In a separate bowl, combine the shredded lettuce, cherry tomatoes, diced avocado, lime juice, salt, and pepper. Toss gently to combine.

6. Divide the lettuce mixture into bowls and top with the chicken fajita mixture.

7. Serve the chicken fajita bowl with a side of guacamole and enjoy!

Nutritional Information:

- Calories: 350

- Protein: 30g

- Carbohydrates: 15g

- Fat: 18g

- Fiber: 8g

Baked Cod with Grilled Zucchini and Wild Rice

Description: This delightful dish features tender baked cod fillets paired with grilled zucchini and fluffy wild rice. It's a light and flavorful combination that will impress your taste buds.

Ingredients:

- 2 cod fillets

- 2 medium zucchini, sliced lengthwise

- 1 tablespoon olive oil

- 1 teaspoon garlic powder

- Salt and pepper to taste

- 1 cup wild rice, cooked according to package instructions

Instructions:

1. Preheat the oven to 400°F (200°C) and line a baking sheet with parchment paper.

2. Place the cod fillets on the prepared baking sheet and drizzle with olive oil. Season with garlic powder, salt, and pepper.

3. Bake the cod fillets for 12-15 minutes until they are opaque and flake easily with a fork.

4. While the cod is baking, heat a grill pan over medium-high heat.

5. Brush the zucchini slices with olive oil and season with salt and pepper.

6. Grill the zucchini slices for 2-3 minutes on each side until they are tender and have grill marks.

7. Serve the baked cod with grilled zucchini and a side of cooked wild rice.

Nutritional Information:

- Calories: 300
- Protein: 25g
- Carbohydrates: 25g
- Fat: 10g
- Fiber: 5g

Vegetable Omelet with Spinach, Mushrooms, and Onions

Description: Start your day with a nutritious and flavorful vegetable omelet filled with fresh spinach, savory mushrooms, and aromatic onions. This satisfying dish is packed with protein and vitamins to fuel your morning.

Ingredients:

- 4 large eggs
- 1 cup fresh spinach, chopped
- 1/2 cup mushrooms, sliced
- 1/4 cup onion, diced
- 1 tablespoon olive oil
- Salt and pepper to taste

Instructions:

1. In a bowl, beat the eggs until well mixed. Season with salt and pepper.
2. Heat olive oil in a non-stick skillet over medium heat.
3. Add the diced onions and sliced mushrooms to the skillet. Sauté until the vegetables are tender.
4. Add the chopped spinach to the skillet and cook until wilted.
5. Pour the beaten eggs over the vegetables in the skillet. Allow the omelet to cook for a few minutes until the edges start to set.
6. Gently lift the edges of the omelet with a spatula to allow the uncooked eggs to flow underneath.
7. Once the omelet is mostly set, carefully flip it over to cook the other side for an additional minute.
8. Slide the omelet onto a plate and fold it in half.
9. Serve the vegetable omelet hot with a side of mixed greens and avocado slices.

Nutritional Information:

- Calories: 250
- Protein: 15g
- Carbohydrates: 8g
- Fat: 18g
- Fiber: 3g

Grilled Chicken Skewers with Bell Peppers and Onions served with a side of Quinoa Salad

Description: Enjoy a delightful and healthy meal with

these grilled chicken skewers featuring colorful bell peppers and onions. Served alongside a refreshing quinoa salad, this dish is bursting with flavors and nutrients.

Ingredients:

- 2 boneless, skinless chicken breasts, cut into chunks
- 1 red bell pepper, cut into chunks
- 1 yellow bell pepper, cut into chunks
- 1 green bell pepper, cut into chunks
- 1 onion, cut into chunks
- Wooden skewers, soaked in water for 30 minutes
- 2 tablespoons olive oil
- 1 tablespoon lemon juice
- 1 teaspoon garlic powder
- Salt and pepper to taste

Quinoa Salad Ingredients:

- 1 cup cooked quinoa
- 1 cucumber, diced
- 1 tomato, diced
- 1/4 cup red onion, finely chopped
- 2 tablespoons fresh parsley, chopped
- Juice of 1 lemon
- 2 tablespoons olive oil
- Salt and pepper to taste

Instructions:

1. Preheat the grill to medium-high heat.

2. Thread the chicken chunks, bell pepper chunks, and onion chunks onto the soaked wooden skewers, alternating the ingredients.

3. In a small bowl, whisk together the olive oil, lemon juice, garlic powder, salt, and pepper. Brush the marinade over the chicken skewers.

4. Place the skewers on the preheated grill and cook for about 10-12 minutes, turning occasionally, until the chicken is cooked through and the vegetables are tender.

5. Meanwhile, in a large bowl, combine the cooked quinoa, diced cucumber, diced tomato, finely chopped red onion, and fresh parsley for the quinoa salad.

6. In a separate small bowl, whisk together the lemon juice, olive oil, salt, and pepper. Drizzle the dressing over the quinoa salad and toss gently to combine.

7. Serve the grilled chicken skewers hot with a side of quinoa salad.

Nutritional Information (Chicken Skewers):

- Calories: 300

- Protein: 30g

- Carbohydrates: 12g

- Fat: 12g

- Fiber: 3g

Nutritional Information (Quinoa Salad):

- Calories: 200
- Protein: 5g
- Carbohydrates: 25g
- Fat: 9g
- Fiber: 5g

Baked Turkey Meatballs with Marinara Sauce and a Side of Steamed Broccoli

Description: These baked turkey meatballs are a lean and flavorful alternative to traditional meatballs. Served with a delicious marinara sauce and a side of steamed broccoli, it's a wholesome and satisfying meal.

Ingredients:

- 1 pound ground turkey
- 1/2 cup breadcrumbs
- 1/4 cup grated Parmesan cheese
- 1/4 cup chopped parsley
- 1 egg, lightly beaten
- 2 cloves garlic, minced
- 1 teaspoon dried oregano
- 1/2 teaspoon salt
- 1/4 teaspoon black pepper
- 2 cups marinara sauce
- Steamed broccoli, for serving

Instructions:

1. Preheat the oven to 400°F (200°C) and line a baking sheet with parchment paper.

2. In a large bowl, combine the ground turkey, breadcrumbs, Parmesan cheese, chopped parsley, egg, minced garlic, dried oregano, salt, and black pepper. Mix until well combined.

3. Shape the mixture into meatballs, about 1 inch in diameter, and place them on the prepared baking sheet.

4. Bake the meatballs in the preheated oven for 20-25 minutes, or until they are cooked through and golden brown.

5. While the meatballs are baking, heat the marinara sauce in a saucepan over medium heat until heated through.

6. Serve the baked turkey meatballs with marinara sauce and a side of steamed broccoli.

Nutritional Information:

- Calories: 250
- Protein: 25g
- Carbohydrates: 15g
- Fat: 10g
- Fiber: 3g

Asian-Inspired Shrimp Stir-Fry with Snap Peas, Carrots, and Brown Rice

Description: This Asian-inspired shrimp stir-fry is a delightful combination of succulent shrimp, crisp snap peas, and vibrant carrots. Served over fluffy brown rice, it's a flavorful and wholesome dish that will satisfy your cravings.

Ingredients:

- 1 pound shrimp, peeled and deveined
- 1 cup snap peas
- 1 cup carrot sticks
- 1 bell pepper, sliced
- 2 cloves garlic, minced
- 1 tablespoon grated ginger
- 2 tablespoons soy sauce
- 1 tablespoon hoisin sauce
- 1 tablespoon sesame oil
- 1 tablespoon vegetable oil
- Cooked brown rice, for serving

Instructions:

1. In a small bowl, whisk together the soy sauce, hoisin sauce, and sesame oil. Set aside.

2. Heat the vegetable oil in a large skillet or wok over medium-high heat.

3. Add the minced garlic and grated ginger to the skillet and sauté for about 1 minute until fragrant.

4. Add the shrimp to the skillet and cook until they turn pink and are cooked through. Remove the shrimp from the skillet and set aside.

5. In the same skillet, add the snap peas, carrot sticks, and bell pepper slices. Stir-fry for about 3-4 minutes until the vegetables are crisp-tender.

6. Return the cooked shrimp to the skillet and pour the sauce mixture over the ingredients. Stir well

to coat everything evenly.

7. Cook for an additional 2-3 minutes until the sauce thickens slightly.

8. Serve the Asian-inspired shrimp stir-fry over cooked brown rice.

Nutritional Information:

- Calories: 300

- Protein: 25g

- Carbohydrates: 30g

- Fat: 10g

- Fiber: 5g

Roasted Pork Tenderloin with Roasted Brussels Sprouts and a Side of Mashed Sweet Potatoes

Description: Indulge in a comforting and flavorful meal with this roasted pork tenderloin served alongside roasted Brussels sprouts and creamy mashed sweet potatoes. This dish is perfect for a hearty dinner that will satisfy your taste buds.

Ingredients:

- 1 pound pork tenderloin

- 1 pound Brussels sprouts, trimmed and halved

- 2 tablespoons olive oil

- 1 tablespoon balsamic vinegar

- 1 teaspoon dried rosemary

- Salt and pepper to taste

- 2 large sweet potatoes, peeled and cubed

- 2 tablespoons butter
- 1/4 cup milk
- Salt and pepper to taste

Instructions:

1. Preheat the oven to 400°F (200°C).

2. Place the pork tenderloin on a baking sheet and season it with salt, pepper, and dried rosemary. Drizzle with olive oil and balsamic vinegar.

3. In a separate bowl, toss the halved Brussels sprouts with olive oil, salt, and pepper.

4. Arrange the seasoned pork tenderloin and Brussels sprouts on the baking sheet, making sure they are spaced apart.

5. Roast in the preheated oven for 20-25 minutes or until the pork reaches an internal temperature of 145°F (63°C) and the Brussels sprouts are tender and slightly caramelized.

6. While the pork and Brussels sprouts are roasting, cook the cubed sweet potatoes in a pot of boiling water until tender, about 15-20 minutes.

7. Drain the cooked sweet potatoes and return them to the pot.

8. Add butter, milk, salt, and pepper to the pot with the sweet potatoes. Mash until smooth and creamy.

9. Slice the roasted pork tenderloin and serve it with the roasted Brussels sprouts and a side of mashed sweet potatoes.

Nutritional Information:

- Calories: 350
- Protein: 25g
- Carbohydrates: 30g
- Fat: 15g
- Fiber: 8g

Lemon Herb Grilled Salmon with a Side of Sautéed Kale and Wild Rice

Description: Elevate your dinner with this refreshing lemon herb grilled salmon served alongside sautéed kale and fluffy wild rice. This dish offers a perfect balance of flavors and nutrients for a wholesome and satisfying meal.

Ingredients:

- 1 pound salmon fillets
- Juice of 1 lemon
- Zest of 1 lemon
- 2 tablespoons chopped fresh herbs (such as dill, parsley, or basil)
- Salt and pepper to taste
- 2 tablespoons olive oil
- 1 bunch kale, stems removed and leaves chopped
- 2 cloves garlic, minced
- Cooked wild rice, for serving

Instructions:

1. Preheat the grill to medium-high heat.
2. In a small bowl, combine the lemon juice, lemon zest, chopped fresh herbs, salt, and pepper.

3. Brush the salmon fillets with olive oil and then generously coat them with the lemon herb mixture.

4. Place the salmon fillets on the preheated grill, skin-side down, and cook for about 4-5 minutes per side, or until the salmon is cooked to your desired level of doneness.

5. While the salmon is grilling, heat olive oil in a large skillet over medium heat.

6. Add the minced garlic to the skillet and sauté for about 1 minute until fragrant.

7. Add the chopped kale leaves to the skillet and sauté until wilted and tender, about 5-7 minutes.

8. Season the sautéed kale with salt and pepper to taste.

9. Serve the lemon herb grilled salmon with a side of sautéed kale and cooked wild rice.

Nutritional Information:

- Calories: 400

- Protein: 30g

- Carbohydrates: 30g

- Fat: 20g

- Fiber: 5g

Spicy Beef Lettuce Wraps filled with Lean Ground Beef, Diced Vegetables, and Served with a Side of Brown Rice

Description: These spicy beef lettuce wraps are a delicious and healthy option for a flavorful meal. Lean ground beef is seasoned with spices, mixed with diced vegetables, and served in crisp lettuce leaves. Accompanied by a side of fluffy brown rice, it's a satisfying dish that packs a punch.

Ingredients:

- 1 pound lean ground beef
- 1 tablespoon vegetable oil
- 1 onion, finely diced
- 2 cloves garlic, minced
- 1 red bell pepper, finely diced
- 1 jalapeño pepper, seeded and minced
- 2 teaspoons chili powder
- 1 teaspoon ground cumin
- 1/2 teaspoon paprika
- Salt and pepper to taste
- Lettuce leaves (such as Bibb or iceberg) for wrapping
- Cooked brown rice, for serving

Instructions:

1. Heat the vegetable oil in a large skillet over medium heat.

2. Add the diced onion and minced garlic to the skillet and sauté until fragrant and translucent.

3. Add the ground beef to the skillet and cook, breaking it up with a spatula, until browned and cooked through.

4. Stir in the diced red bell pepper, minced jalapeño pepper, chili powder, ground cumin, paprika, salt,

and pepper. Cook for an additional 3-4 minutes to allow the flavors to meld together.

5. Remove the skillet from heat and let the beef mixture cool slightly.

6. Spoon the spicy beef mixture onto lettuce leaves and wrap them up like tacos.

7. Serve the spicy beef lettuce wraps with a side of cooked brown rice.

Nutritional Information:

- Calories: 350

- Protein: 25g

- Carbohydrates: 30g

- Fat: 12g

- Fiber: 5g

Grilled Shrimp and Vegetable Kebabs with a Side of Cauliflower Rice

Description: Enjoy a light and flavorful meal with these grilled shrimp and vegetable kebabs. Skewered with colorful vegetables and succulent shrimp, these kebabs are bursting with taste. Served alongside cauliflower rice, it's a low-carb and satisfying dish that's perfect for a wholesome dinner.

Ingredients:

- 1 pound shrimp, peeled and deveined

- 1 red bell pepper, cut into chunks

- 1 yellow bell pepper, cut into chunks

- 1 zucchini, sliced into rounds

- 1 red onion, cut into chunks
- 2 tablespoons olive oil
- 2 cloves garlic, minced
- 1 teaspoon paprika
- Salt and pepper to taste
- Cauliflower rice, for serving

Instructions:

1. Preheat the grill to medium-high heat.
2. In a bowl, combine the olive oil, minced garlic, paprika, salt, and pepper.
3. Thread the shrimp, bell pepper chunks, zucchini slices, and red onion chunks onto skewers.
4. Brush the kebabs with the olive oil mixture, coating them evenly.
5. Place the kebabs on the preheated grill and cook for 2-3 minutes per side, or until the shrimp is cooked through and the vegetables are slightly charred.
6. While the kebabs are grilling, prepare the cauliflower rice according to the package instructions.
7. Serve the grilled shrimp and vegetable kebabs with a side of cauliflower rice.

Nutritional Information:

- Calories: 300
- Protein: 25g
- Carbohydrates: 15g

- Fat: 15g

- Fiber: 5g

Baked Chicken Thighs with Roasted Root Vegetables and Quinoa

Description: Treat yourself to a wholesome and flavorful meal with these baked chicken thighs accompanied by roasted root vegetables and a side of nutritious quinoa. The chicken thighs are tender and juicy, while the roasted vegetables add a delicious depth of flavor. Combined with quinoa, this dish is a complete and satisfying dinner option.

Ingredients:

- 4 bone-in, skin-on chicken thighs

- 1 tablespoon olive oil

- 1 teaspoon dried thyme

- 1 teaspoon dried rosemary

- Salt and pepper to taste

- 2 carrots, peeled and chopped

- 2 parsnips, peeled and chopped

- 2 beets, peeled and chopped

- 2 tablespoons balsamic vinegar

- 1 tablespoon honey

- 1 cup cooked quinoa

Instructions:

1. Preheat the oven to 400°F (200°C).

2. Place the chicken thighs in a baking dish and drizzle them with olive oil. Season with dried

thyme, dried rosemary, salt, and pepper. Rub the seasoning into the chicken thighs.

3. In a separate bowl, toss the chopped carrots, parsnips, and beets with olive oil, balsamic vinegar, honey, salt, and pepper.

4. Arrange the seasoned chicken thighs and the mixed vegetables on a baking sheet, making sure they are spread out evenly.

5. Bake in the preheated oven for 30-35 minutes, or until the chicken thighs are cooked through and the vegetables are tender and caramelized.

6. While the chicken and vegetables are baking, prepare the quinoa according to the package instructions.

7. Serve the baked chicken thighs with the roasted root vegetables and a side of cooked quinoa.

Nutritional Information:

- Calories: 400
- Protein: 25g
- Carbohydrates: 30g
- Fat: 20g
- Fiber: 6g

Spinach and Mushroom Frittata with a Side of Mixed Greens and Avocado Slices

Description: Start your day with a nutritious and delicious spinach and mushroom frittata served alongside a bed of mixed greens and slices of creamy avocado. This frittata is packed with flavor and nutrients, making it a perfect choice for a satisfying breakfast or brunch.

Ingredients:

- 6 large eggs
- 1 tablespoon olive oil
- 1 small onion, diced
- 8 ounces mushrooms, sliced
- 2 cups baby spinach
- Salt and pepper to taste
- Mixed greens, for serving
- 1 avocado, sliced

Instructions:

1. Preheat the oven to 350°F (175°C).
2. In a mixing bowl, whisk the eggs until well beaten. Set aside.
3. Heat olive oil in a skillet over medium heat. Add the diced onion and sauté until translucent.
4. Add the sliced mushrooms to the skillet and cook until they release their moisture and become tender.
5. Add the baby spinach to the skillet and cook until wilted. Season with salt and pepper to taste.
6. Pour the beaten eggs over the cooked vegetables in the skillet. Stir gently to combine.
7. Transfer the skillet to the preheated oven and bake for 15-20 minutes, or until the frittata is set and lightly golden.
8. While the frittata is baking, arrange a bed of mixed greens on a serving platter and top with

slices of avocado.

9. Remove the frittata from the oven and let it cool slightly before slicing into wedges.

10. Serve the spinach and mushroom frittata on the bed of mixed greens with avocado slices on the side.

Nutritional Information:

- Calories: 250

- Protein: 15g

- Carbohydrates: 10g

- Fat: 18g

- Fiber: 5g

Grilled Chicken Skewers with Bell Peppers and Onions, Served with a Side of Quinoa Salad

Description: These grilled chicken skewers are a delicious and colorful dish that combines tender chicken with vibrant bell peppers and onions. Served with a refreshing quinoa salad, it's a well-balanced and satisfying meal option.

Ingredients:

- 1 pound chicken breast, cut into bite-sized cubes

- 1 red bell pepper, cut into chunks

- 1 green bell pepper, cut into chunks

- 1 yellow bell pepper, cut into chunks

- 1 red onion, cut into chunks

- 2 tablespoons olive oil

- 2 cloves garlic, minced

- 1 teaspoon paprika
- 1 teaspoon dried oregano
- Salt and pepper to taste
- Wooden skewers, soaked in water

Instructions:

1. Preheat the grill to medium-high heat.
2. In a bowl, combine the olive oil, minced garlic, paprika, dried oregano, salt, and pepper.
3. Thread the chicken pieces, bell pepper chunks, and onion chunks onto the soaked wooden skewers, alternating between the ingredients.
4. Brush the chicken skewers with the olive oil mixture, coating them evenly.
5. Place the skewers on the preheated grill and cook for about 10-12 minutes, turning occasionally, until the chicken is cooked through and the vegetables are slightly charred.
6. While the skewers are grilling, prepare the quinoa salad by combining cooked quinoa with diced vegetables of your choice, such as cucumbers, cherry tomatoes, and fresh herbs. Toss with a light dressing of olive oil, lemon juice, salt, and pepper.
7. Serve the grilled chicken skewers with bell peppers and onions alongside the quinoa salad.

Nutritional Information:

- Calories: 350
- Protein: 30g

- Carbohydrates: 25g

- Fat: 12g

- Fiber: 5g

Baked Turkey Meatballs with Marinara Sauce and a Side of Steamed Broccoli

Description: These baked turkey meatballs are a healthier twist on a classic comfort food. Tender and flavorful, they are served with a delicious marinara sauce and accompanied by steamed broccoli for a nutritious and satisfying meal.

Ingredients:

- 1 pound ground turkey

- 1/2 cup breadcrumbs

- 1/4 cup grated Parmesan cheese

- 1/4 cup chopped fresh parsley

- 1 egg, lightly beaten

- 2 cloves garlic, minced

- 1 teaspoon dried oregano

- Salt and pepper to taste

- 2 cups marinara sauce

- Steamed broccoli, for serving

Instructions:

1. Preheat the oven to 375°F (190°C).

2. In a large bowl, combine ground turkey, breadcrumbs, grated Parmesan cheese, chopped parsley, minced garlic, dried oregano, salt, and pepper. Mix well until all ingredients are evenly

incorporated.

3. Shape the mixture into meatballs, about 1 inch in diameter, and place them on a baking sheet lined with parchment paper.

4. Bake the meatballs in the preheated oven for 20-25 minutes, or until they are cooked through and golden brown.

5. While the meatballs are baking, heat the marinara sauce in a saucepan over medium heat until warmed through.

6. Once the meatballs are cooked, transfer them to the marinara sauce and simmer for a few minutes to allow the flavors to meld together.

7. Serve the baked turkey meatballs with marinara sauce alongside steamed broccoli.

Nutritional Information:

- Calories: 300
- Protein: 25g
- Carbohydrates: 15g
- Fat: 10g
- Fiber: 5g